I AM ...
YOUTHING!

A Presentation by Tamara D. Savino

About the Five Tibetan Rites: Exercises for Healing, Rejuvenation, and Longevity.

& Ancient Secret of the Fountain of Youth, Book 2

A Pocket Full of Wisdom by Tamara Savino (Author)

Preface

Hidden in the high Himalayas 2,500 years ago, Tibetan Lamas developed five simple range of motion exercises they called "Rites." These Rites have remarkable powers of rejuvenation; indeed, they have rightfully been called a "Fountain of Youth."

Actual reported benefits from the Five Rites are legion. They include:

- greater energy
- increased sex drive
- a more youthful appearance
- diminished grey hair
- hair regrowth
- weight loss
- improved eyesight
- better memory
- enhanced sense of well-being
- longer life

The Five Rites are comparatively easy to practice and can be performed in 15 - 30 minutes. The cost-benefit ratio is rather favorable.

In 1939, Peter Kelder published *The Eye of Revelation*, a small book which revealed the Tibetan Rites of Rejuvenation to the West.   He republished it in 1946 with new information, but both editions were nearly lost. While the originals were languishing, millions of reprint copies were sold under the titles:

- *The Five Rites of Rejuvenation*" (Borderland Sciences, 1969)
- *The Ancient Secret of the Fountain of Youth* (Harbor Press, 1985)

In more recent years, newer editions were published:

- *The Five Tibetans by Christopher S. Kilham (Healing Arts Press, 1994)*
- *The 10-Minute Rejuvenation Plan by Carolinda Witt, (Three Rivers Press, 2007)*
- *The Eye of Revelation: The Ancient Tibetan Rites of Rejuvenation edited by J. Watt (Booklocker, 2008).*

Some were faithful to Kelder's original texts, most were not. The Borderland Science's editions and the Booklocker edition are faithful renditions of the 1939 and 1946 editions of the *Eye of Revelation*.

Tamara Savino's Presentation "I AM YOUTHING" ... Is all about sharing the Five Tibetan Rites of Rejuvenation: the history, practice, theories about how and why they work, where to find more information and support. The Five Rights of Rejuvenation tells the fascinating story of how a mysterious Colonel Bradford (Major-General Sir Wilfrid Malleson) discovered the Five Rites in a Tibetan monastery and brought them to the West. His friend, Peter Kelder, published them in 1939 and republished them in 1946.

Perhaps the most interesting thing is that James Hilton, author of Lost Horizon, had a hand in bringing the Five Rites to the West. Hilton's story is about a secret Tibetan monastery hidden in the Himalayas where life extension is practiced, a monastery called Shangri-La. Have you ever heard of Shangri-La. You're about to experience it in Part II (the Exercises) in this two part Presentation.

Purpose

In 2008, I purchased an original copy of Peter Kelder's 1946 edition of the *Eye of Revelation* with no other thought than to simply enjoy owning a scarce copy of a book that was important to me.

No book can survive forever unless it is continuously and accurately republished. Today there are only two known surviving copies of the 1939 edition. And just one of the 1946. Without these originals, Kelder's true work might have been lost forever. I was blessed to be led to this Exercise Regmin years ago and decided to publish this two Part Presentation: "I AM YOUTHING" – to help others enjoy increased energy and experience optimal well-ness.

My purpose is to find ways to preserve Peter Kelder's authentic message and share it with all of YOU! The exercises are fun and easy to perform and you will quickly enjoy the "YOUTHING" process! Yet, no one will ever know or understand these Rites better than Peter Kelder, Colonel Bradford or even the Tibetan lamas who created them. Have fun with it! Ok, let's get started!

Recite Aloud: "I … AM … YOUTHING!"

PETER KELDERS – THE EYE OF REVELATION
The Five Tibetan Rites of Rejuvenation – "I AM … Youthing." Presented by Tamara Savino

The Five Tibetan Rites: Exercises for Healing, Rejuvenation, and Longevity

"I AM YOUTHING." A PRESENTATION By Tamara D. Savino

Background

In 1985 a book called **The Ancient Secret of the Fountain of Youth** written by **Peter Kelder** was published which for the first time fully described an exercise program for "Youthing". This is an exercise program used by Tibetan monks to live long, vibrant and healthy lives. In fact, this book states that many have lived longer than most can imagine by following the program often called the "Five Tibetan Rites". The benefits are described in this book and a subsequent book 2 with an expanded description of the program by the publisher called the **Ancient Secret of the Fountain of Youth - Book 2**, a companion to the original book by Peter Kelder. Many thanks to the *Publisher Doubleday* for such a special an expanded explanation of the Five Rites.

Potential Benefits of the Five Rites

The authors provide many examples of the benefits of the "Five Tibetan Rites" including the following: looking much younger; sleeping soundly; waking up feeling refreshed and energetic; release from serious medical problems including difficulties with spines; relief from problems with joints; release from pain; better memory; arthritis relief; weight loss; improved vision; youthing instead of aging; greatly improved physical strength, endurance and vigor; improved emotional and mental health; enhanced sense of well-being and harmony; and very high overall energy.

How the Five Rites Work

Medical professions explain the benefits based on their personal perspective and I suggest you read the entire two books for a broad overview. However, the majority share the view that the rites represent a system of exercise that affects the body, emotions and mind. The Tibetans claim that these exercises activate and stimulate the seven key chakras that in turn stimulate all the glands of the endocrine system. The endocrine system is responsible for the body's overall functioning and aging process. This means that the Five Rites will affect the functioning of all your organs and systems, including the physical and energetic systems and that includes the aging process. The man who brought these Five Rights out of Tibet stated that "performing the Five Rites stimulates the circulation of essential life energy throughout the body".

Chakras

Chakra is an Indian Sanskrit word that translates to mean "Wheel of Spinning Energy". Chakras are spinning wheels or vortexes of energy of different color that perform many functions connecting our energy fields, bodies and the Cosmic Energy Field. Chakras are powerful electrical and magnetic fields. Chakras govern the endocrine system that in turn regulates all of the body's functions including the ageing process. Energy flows from the Universal Energy Field through the chakras into the energy systems within our bodies, including the Meridian System.

Our bodies contain seven major chakras or energy centers and 122 minor chakras. The major chakras are located at the base of the spine (Root Chakra), at the navel (Sacral Chakra), in the solar plexus (Solar Plexus Chakra), within your heart (Heart Chakra), within the throat (Throat Chakra), at the center of your forehead (Brow or Third Eye Chakra), and at the top of your head (Crown Chakra). These chakras are linked together with all other energy systems in the body and various layers of the auras.

The Speed of the chakra spin is a key to vibrant health. The other keys to vibrant health that relates to the chakra is ensuring they are clear of negative energy and that they are perfectly shaped and not distorted.

The Five Rites speed up the spinning of the chakras, coordinate their spin so they are in complete harmony, distribute pure Prana energy to the endocrine system, and in turn to all organs and processes in the body. This is one of the major requirements for vibrant health, rejuvenation and youthfulness.

The Five Rites Exercise Program

This program is often described as a modified yoga program. Simply put, yoga is a science that unites the body, mind and spirit. Today this is often called Mind/ Body Healing. The author of the book believes that yoga was brought to Tibet from India in the 11th or 12th century and that Tibetan monks over time developed modified these exercises and developed an effective program of exercises that western society now calls the "Five Tibetan Rites". The rugged mountainous conditions these monks live in may well account for their particular emphasis on vigor. Many of the yoga exercises and practices being taught in the western world today are very new. The "Five Tibetan Rites" are exactly what the ancient Tibetans developed over many centuries of time. Therefore it's very important to do the "Five Tibetan Rites" exactly as they are presented without altering the form or sequence to achieve some of the benefits accrued to these "Rites".

Beginning the "Five Rites" Exercise Program

1. For the first week, and only if you are relatively healthy and fit, do each exercise three times.
2. If you are inactive, overweight, or have health problems begin these exercises doing one of the first three each day, and only if you feel totally comfortable doing this. Later in this article I will describe exercises you can do to help yourself strengthen so you can begin to do the "Five Rites". If you have any concerns whatsoever, please consult with your physician. Individuals on serious medications should consult with their physicians.
3. If you are overweight do not do Rites #4 and #5 until you have developed some strength and endurance. Do the substitutes for #4 and #5 until you yourself feel ready to begin doing #4 and #5 of the "Five Rites".
4. Do only what you feel comfortable doing. That may be only one of each exercise for the first week. Build up to two of each exercise the second week, three of each exercise the third week, etc. or at a faster pace only if your body does not hurt when you do these exercises.
5. 21 is the maximum of each exercise you should ever do. If you want to enhance your program, do the exercises at a faster pace, but do not so more than 21 of each exercise each day. Doing more than 21 repetitions of each exercise in any day will affect your chakras negatively and can create imbalances in your body.
6. The "Five Rites" may stimulate detoxification and often creates many unpleasant physical symptoms. This is why it's recommended to increase the number of each exercise gradually on a weekly basis. I also recommend a vibrational detoxification with Essences. For more information on vibrational detoxification with Essences please visit my website **www.tamarasavino.com**.
7. If you have not exercised for some time, prepare to begin your "Five Rites" exercise program by walking daily, for a

half hour each day if possible. Another alternative in preparation for the Five Rites is a stretching program with a gradual increase in the types of stretching exercises and the duration of this program.

8. A sugar free and low fat diet is an important support when integrating the "Five Rites" exercise program into your life. Also check for Digestive Food Sensitivities and eliminate all foods you do not digest easily.

9. Do the Five Rites exercises every day. The maximum you should skip is one day each week. If the exercises are done less than six days each week, the results will be greatly reduced.

10. If on certain days your time is limited, do 3 repetitions of each exercise. This takes less than five minutes.

11. For maximum benefit, do the exercises before breakfast in the morning, if at all possible. If this is not possible do them anytime during the day.

Detoxification

Detoxification is a process that helps to clean out of the physical and energetic body toxins or poisons that have accumulated in your physical cells, organs, systems and in your energetic systems (auras, chakras, meridian system and all electromagnetic, magnetic and electric systems). I strongly recommend that people beginning the "Five Rites" exercise program undertake an Essence detoxification program either before or as they begin these exercises.

If you have never detoxified you will probably have many poisons accumulated in your body and energetic systems. A full detoxification program with Flower Essence, Gem Essences, and Tree Essences will eliminate all toxins. Detoxifying with Essences uses vibrational essences, or what is sometimes called vibrational medicine to clear your systems of toxins and poisons. This includes the elimination of parasites, candida, viruses, and all poisons from pollution, pesticides etc.

This vibrational approach to detoxification is completely complementary to the exercises of the "Five Rites". Detoxification is essential for vibrant and long life. For more information please refer to my article "Detoxification with Essences" and other vibrational health articles on My Website at:

www.tamarasavino.com

"Five Tibetan Rites" Exercise Program

The following instructions and photographs for the "Five Rites" and other preparatory exercises as taken from the book Ancient Secret of the Fountain of Youth, Book 2. I will show the exact Five Rights exercises, a group of exercises for those who need to develop flexibility and strength before beginning to do the "Five Rites", and a set of warm-up exercises. I strongly recommend you purchase the book (eventually) since it provides detailed information about methodology, concerns and benefits not included in this article.

SPECIAL CAUTION: Spinning and stretching through the following exercises can aggravate certain health conditions such as any type of heart problem, multiple sclerosis, Parkinsons's Disease, severe arthritis of the spine, uncontrolled high blood pressure, a hyperthyroid condition, or vertigo. Problems may also be caused if you are taking drugs that cause dizziness. Please consult your physician prior to beginning ANY/ALL exercises, especially this Exercise Regimen.

The Five Tibetan Rites

Rite #1 Stand erect with arms outstretched horizontal to the floor, palms facing down. Your arms should be in line with your shoulders. Spin around clockwise until you become slightly dizzy. Gradually increase number of spins from 1 spin to 21 spins.

Breathing: Inhale and exhale deeply as you do the spins.

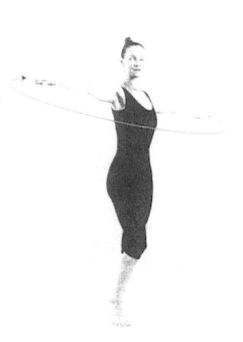

Rite #2 Lie flat on the floor, face up. Fully extend your arms Along your sides and place the palms of your hands against the floor, keeping fingers close together. Then raise your head off the floor tucking your chin into your chest. As you do this, lift your legs, knees straight, into a vertical position. If possible, extend the legs over the body towards your head. Do not let the knees bend. Then slowly lower the legs and head to the floor, always Keeping the knees straight. Allow the muscles to relax, and repeat.

Breathing: Breathe in deeply as you lift your head and legs and exhale as you lower your head and legs.

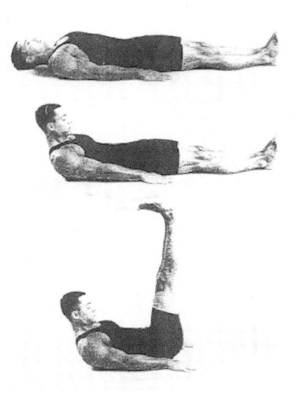

Rite #3 Kneel on the floor with the body erect. The hands should be placed on the backs of your thigh muscles. Incline the head and neck forward, tucking your chin in against your chest. Then throw the head and neck backward, arching the spine. Your toes should be curled under through this exercise. As you arch, you will brace your arms and hands against the thighs for support. After the arching return your body to an erect position and begin the rite all over again.

Breathing: Inhale as you arch the spine and exhale as you return to an erect position.

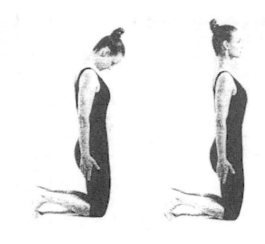

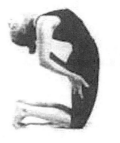

Rite #4 Sit down on the floor with your legs straight out in front of you and your feet about 12" apart. With the trunk of the body erect, place the palms of your hands on the floor alongside your buttocks. Then tuck the chin forward against the chest. Now drop the head backward as far as it will go. At the same time raise your body so that the knees bend while the arms remain straight. Then tense every muscle in your body. Finally let the muscles relax as you return to your original sitting position. Rest before repeating this Rite.

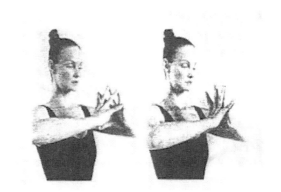

Breathing:

Breathe in as you raise up, hold your breath as you tense the muscles, and breathe out fully as you come down.

Rite #5 Lie down with your face down to the floor. You will be supported by the hands palms down against the floor and the toes in the flexed position. Throughout this rite, the hands and feet should be kept straight. Start with your arms perpendicular to the Floor, and the spine arched, so that the body Is in a sagging position. Now throw the head back as far as possible. The, bending at the hips, bring the body up into an inverted "V". At the same time, bring the chin forward, Tucking it against the chest.

Breathing: Breathe in deeply as you raise the body, and exhale fully as you lower the body.

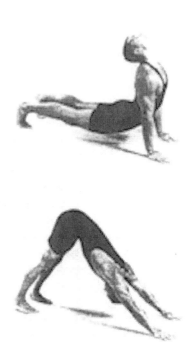

Exercises In Preparation For Doing the Five Tibetan Rites

The following group of exercises has been developed as a preparation for doing the Five Rites, or as an alternative when you are unable to do any of the Five Rites. Doing these exercises will help you strengthen and become more flexible to be able to do the Five Rites as they have been described above.

Do these alternative exercises in the sequence from one to five and when possible, substitute the Five Rite exercise into this alternative program until you have fully integrated the Five Rites.

As with the Five Rites, begin by doing two or three of each exercise daily, until you are able to do 10 each day. Once you are able to do ten of these alternatives, you should be ready to begin doing the Five Rite exercises themselves.

Alternative (for Rite#1)

Exercise #1 Stand with your feet about 12 inches apart. Extend your arms palms down until your arms are level with your shoulders. Swing your arms to the right, letting your slapping your left hand against your right shoulder, with your right hand slapping against the small of your back. Then swing your arms in the opposite direction, having your right hand slap against your left shoulder and the back of your left hand slap against the small of your back. As you swing back and forth allow your torso and legs to follow the movement. Allow your heels to lift from the floor but do not allow either foot to completely leave the floor. As you swing right turn your head right, and turn your head left as you swing to the left.

Breathing: Breathe in rhythm to your swinging Movement.

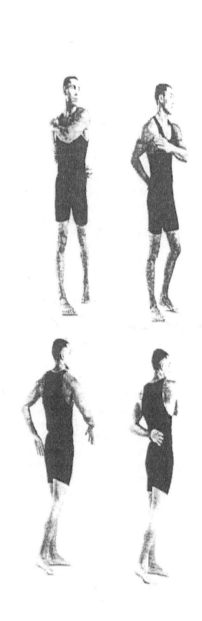

Alternative (for Rite #2) Exercise #2

Lie down on the floor and elevate your head and shoulders propping up on your elbows keeping your forearms flat on the floor, palms facing down. Keeping your legs straight, hold them off the floor For 20 or 30 seconds.**Breathing:** Inhale as you raise your legs, breathe in and out normally while holding your legs up, and exhale as you lower your legs.

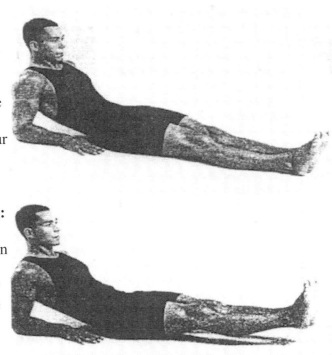

Alternative (for Rite #3) Exercise #3

Stand with your back to the wall and your feet 12 - 18 inches apart. Without moving your feet bend forward from the hips so that your buttocks rest against the wall. Slide downward, bending your knees as you go. Keep sliding down until your thighs are horizontal, as if you were sitting in a chair. Hold this position for 15 seconds and then slide back up.

Breathing: Begin to exhale as you slide down to the chair position

Inhale when you slide back up.

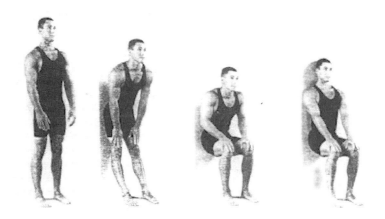

Alternative (for Rite #4) Exercise #4

Lie flat on your back, your arms straight, palms down, feet flat, and knees bent. Press your pelvis up a few inches off the floor and hold it for 10 seconds. Release and lower your pelvis to its original position.

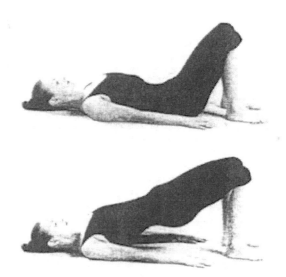

Breathing: Inhale as you lift your pelvis and Exhale as you lower your pelvis.

Alternative (for Rite #5) Exercise #5

Begin in the table position. Curl your toes under And bend your hips raising your buttocks so that Your body forms an inverted "V". Your knees will lift up off the floor, your legs will be straight, and your outstretched arms will be in a straight line with your back. Hold this position for 15 seconds.

Breathing: Inhale as you raise your buttocks, breath Slowly and deeply while holding the position, and exhale as you return to the table position.

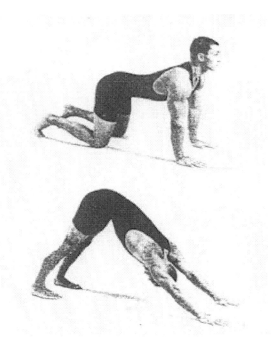

Warm-up Exercises

The following group of exercises has been developed to open, relax, release tension, to strengthen various parts of the body, and to provide toning to different parts of your body.

If you are overweight, in poor physical condition, or experiencing serious illness, this group of exercises is an excellent to help you begin your journey towards physical fitness. I suggest you do these warm-up exercises prior to the Five Rites if you are overweight or have not exercised in a long time.

Begin this group of exercises by doing 2 of each exercise and then gradually increase the repetition until you are able to do 10 of each warm-up exercise.

Warm-Up Exercise #1

Stand upright, tilt your head sideways towards your left shoulder and hold it for five seconds, then tilt your head towards your chest and hold it 5 seconds. Then tilt your head towards your left Shoulder and hold it five seconds, and lastly tilt your head backward and hold it five seconds. Return to a normal position.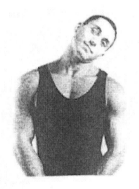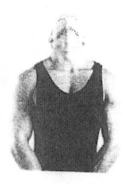

Breathing: Exhale

as you move your head around, and inhale as you return to the upright position.

Warm-Up Exercise #2 Stand upright, slowly rotate your shoulders in a forward circular motion 5 times, then reverse the movement and rotate your shoulders in a backward circular motion 5 times.

Breathing: Breathe normally but deeply as you do this exercise.

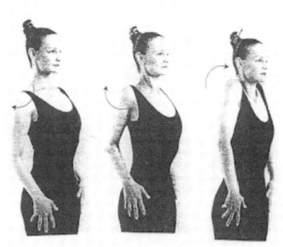

Warm-Up Exercise #3

Stand upright with your arms help up, your elbows bent, and your hands together in front of your chest, with your fingertips touching and palms apart. Press inward on your fingers until their inside surfaces are almost touching. Your palms should not be touching. Release and press your fingers again.

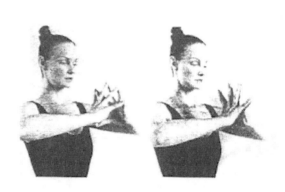

Breathing: Breathe normally.

Warm-Up Exercise #4

In a relaxed standing position, hold your arms in front of you. Clasp your right hand around your left wrist, with your thumb against the inside of the wrist. Squeeze gently but firmly five times. Repeat the procedure with the left hand Squeezing the right wrist.

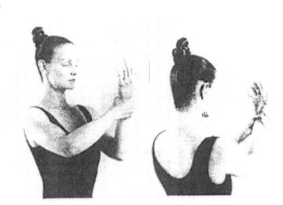

Breathing: Breathe normally.

Warm-Up Exercise #5

Recline on the floor, resting the upper part of your body on your upper arms. Flex your knees and rhythmically bang Them up and down against the floor in rapid succession. Your heels should remain on the floor throughout this exercise. Do this exercise for 20 - 30 seconds.

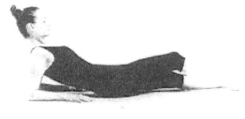

Breathing: Breathe normally through this exercise.

Warm-Up Exercise #6

Get down on the floor on your
hands and Knees with your
hands positioned under your
shoulders and your knees
under your hips. Bring your
chin up and rotate your hips so
the tailbone moves up, arching
your back down. Then tuck
your chin into your chest and
rotate your back so that your
pelvis moves down, arching
you're your back down.

Breathing: Inhale as you
move your tailbone up and
exhale as you move your
tailbone down.

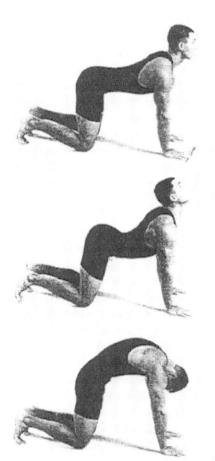

Conclusion: The daily practice of the "YOUTHING" exercises I have described in this Presentation: "I AM YOUTHING" … is an essential element of vibrant health. It's a proven fact that people who lose weight can only maintain their weight loss if they incorporate a daily exercise program into their everyday lives.

These exercises will stretch muscles you haven't felt in years so approach this program gently and begin with one or two repetitions each day, increasing each exercise by one repetition every week. After you are able to do ten repetitions of the Alternate Exercise program, you should be able to begin to do the Five Rites.

And add a half hour of a brisk walk on a daily basis. Not only will it contribute to your physical health, it will give you the opportunity to enjoy all of nature around you. You will feel younger than you have felt in many years.

Happy Youthing! With Love and Peace,

Tamara D. Savino
I AM YOUTHING!
tamarasavino.com

A Pocket Full of Wisdom *2010*

A Pocket Full of Wisdom

A Journey of Rich Proclamations
By Tamara Dawn Savino

A Pocket Full of Wisdom *2010*

About the Author

*Hello, I am Tamara Dawn Savino, an Author who inspires everyone with the faith and purpose of an Advancing Healthy, Joyful, Rich and Abundant Life. A Pocket Full of Wisdom **2010***

About These Rich Proclamations

On average, it takes about twenty to forty days of continuous repetition to establish the Rich Proclamations presented in this book. Best results will be enjoyed as you feel the powerful words take shape and have a belief and take action that you will be blessed. Try reciting these Rich Proclamations aloud with true "Feeling" upon waking and upon sleeping for better results. Not every Proclamation in this book is for "Everyone". So, please choose distinct Proclamations written herein that "resonates" with your being and simply enjoy those. Start small and if necessary, choose only one Proclamation to enjoy before delving into deeper or more spiritually complex Proclamations provided in this manuscript. Each Proclamation speaks to the Present day as IF the Blessing has already taken shape and come to pass. Practice visualizing and feeling the words take shape in your life for better results. There are absolutely no guarantees any person reading this book will become Rich. These proclamations when practiced may yield positive advancements in the life of the person(s) who read it. The Author of A Pocket Full of Wisdom, Amazon.com, Kindle or any other associated Market or Publisher does not accept any liability or responsibility for the outcomes of the study or practices defined in this publication.

Thank you and Rich Blessings, Optimal Health, Joy and Peace to You!

In Love and Light, Tamara.

Tamara Dawn Savino *A Pocket Full of Wisdom*
2010

Forward

It is virtuous to adore, and my true virtue
is my Everlasting Love toward God,
my sons A.J. and Nick, my Family,
Friendships, and Community.

Tamara Dawn Savino A Pocket Full of
Wisdom **2010**

Dedication

I dedicate this book and all of my writing to my amazing sons Anthony J. and Nicholas V. My words are inspired by my love for God and for my sons. God is my giver and gift and my Eternal Abundant and Very Rich Life! *A Pocket Full of Wisdom **2010***

Increase

I apply myself and my capabilities to do all I can do, every day, and do it in a perfectly successful manner; putting the power of success, and the purpose of being rich, into everything that I do! A Pocket Full of Wisdom **2010**

I am enjoying continuous increase, and I'm also giving it with pleasure to all with whom I deal. A Pocket Full of Wisdom

2010

I am a "Creative Center", from which God's increase is given off to all. I am certain of this fact, therefore I convey an assurance of this fact to every man, woman, and child with whom I am acquainted. A Pocket Full of Wisdom **2010**

I am an advancing Rich person that joyfully gives advancement likewise to others along my pathway. A Pocket Full of Wisdom **2010**

Because I feel faithful, I let Faith manifest in every transaction; allowing every act, tone, and expression express the quiet Infinite Spirit's powerful assurance that I am increasing; and that I am already eternally Rich, healthy and happy. A Pocket Full of Wisdom **2010**

My professional and personal business increases rapidly, and I am pleasantly surprised at the unexpected benefits which come to me. A Pocket Full of Wisdom **2010**

There is no competition in my creative mind; "What I want for myself, I want for everybody!" A Pocket Full of Wisdom **2010**

God helps me and the right people and things arrive at just the "Ripe" time in Divine Order so that I may likewise help myself. A Pocket Full of Wisdom **2010**

When any good opportunity to be more than I am now is presented and I feel impelled toward it, I take action and take it. It is the first step toward a greater opportunity and increase. A Pocket Full of Wisdom **2010**

My thoughts are held up upon the creative plane and I have an unlimited supply as I act on the moral level of peaceful and harmonious friendship and fellowship. A Pocket Full of Wisdom **2010**

I tend to the matters of today; sufficient is the day! A Pocket Full of Wisdom **2010**

There are no obstructions or even any appearance of any obstruction at a distance; adverse appearances are false, so they effortlessly vanish as I approach, or Spirit paves a new way for me. *A Pocket Full of Wisdom* **2010**

I disallow any or all anxious thoughts to possible disasters, obstacles, panics, or unfavorable combinations of circumstances; I am provided a good and swift route to overcome victoriously! A Pocket Full of Wisdom **2010**

Even if others are having hard times or poor business, Conversely, Time after time I easily find great opportunities as I bless and increase those along my pathway! A Pocket Full of Wisdom **2010**

I think of and look upon my world as a something which is becoming; I am ever-increasing and affluent. I live in an ever-increasing and affluent Rich and Happy Life now! A Pocket Full of Wisdom **2010**

I readily speak in terms of advancement, about things that are becoming, and increasing! I am living an ever-increasing and an affluent Rich and Happy Life now! A Pocket Full of Wisdom **2010**

I am always encouraged about Supreme protection, provisions, and pardon. A Pocket Full of Wisdom **2010**

When I desire to have a certain thing at a certain time; it arrives in Divine Order, just on time! A Pocket Full of Wisdom **2010**

If I do not receive a thing, it is not for me. If it is good for me, I receive it or its equivalent; or something much greater! A Pocket Full of Wisdom **2010**

I'm incredibly faithful as I hold to my purpose, have gratitude, and do the most and the best I can do daily! A Pocket Full of Wisdom **2010**

I am successful because I possess and further develop the necessary talents to do what I desire; all the while, enjoying the doing of my work. A Pocket Full of Wisdom

2010

I apply my capabilities and talents and keep right on course, so when I approach a place, a natural ability is furnished. A Pocket Full of Wisdom **2010**

I am in full harmony with God as I lively entertain a sincere gratitude for Supreme
Blessings I receive now! A Pocket Full of Wisdom **2010**

By thought, the things I desire manifest; by faith and action I receive it, it's equivalent or greater! A Pocket Full of Wisdom **2010**

I prepare for the reception of what I desire, and I begin now. I am free, living a Rich and Happy Life now! A Pocket Full of Wisdom **2010**

I enjoy the free and unrestricted use of all the things which may be necessary to my fullest mental, spiritual, and physical enfoldment. A Pocket Full of Wisdom **2010**

I gracefully and humbly go before God and give Gratitude and Thanksgiving for the Eternal Purse of the Spirit of God is pouring an endless Waterfall of Prosperity over me! A Pocket Full of Wisdom **2010**

I activate now, my desire for a richer, fuller, and more abundant life; that blesses me with good health, great wealth, true love, faith, and gratitude! A Pocket Full of Wisdom **2010**

I live a real happy life; real life reaches a more complete expression of all that I can give forth through my body, mind, and soul.
A Pocket Full of Wisdom **2010**

I am established in happiness and Godly Love;

My heart is now free, open, and happily living true love!

I easily give and receive God's Divine Love with poise and grace in the most wonderful ways! A Pocket Full of Wisdom **2010**

I am an irresistible magnet for goodness, love, wealth, and health! A Pocket Full of Wisdom **2010**

I now rise to my greatest possible height in talent and soul development. A Pocket Full of Wisdom **2010**

I now have plenty of money, to unfold my soul and further develop all of my talents and capabilities to the fullest expression of life! A Pocket Full of Wisdom **2010**

I am easily and effortlessly provided many resources to use in love and understanding, and I am provided a way to acquire plenty of money to buy them with. I use these resources wisely according to the Divine Plan. A Pocket Full of Wisdom **2010**

I am wholly aligned with the purpose of nature and its advancement and unfolding life for me; I shall now have all that contributes to the Supreme power, elegance, beauty, and richness of my life and for the lives of those I truly Love. A Pocket Full of Wisdom **2010**

I am a balanced Rich person with sound mind, body and spirit – all correctly aligned and I'm optimally healthy and happy! A Pocket Full of Wisdom **2010**

I am living a real life with the complete expression of all that I can give forth through my body, mind, and soul for myself, my family. A Pocket Full of Wisdom **2010**

I am responsible with money; I'm unconcerned with money going out. As my money circulates it is multiplied; I receive more cash, colorful wealth-building checks, and surprising lavish gifts with ease. A Pocket Full of Wisdom **2010**

Everything I need, desire or require that is good for me is provided easily and effortlessly from the Supreme, just on time!A Pocket Full of Wisdom **2010**

I am living a gloriously happy and satisfied life; I'm living fully in every function and capacity now, and the same is true of my mind and soul. A Pocket Full of Wisdom **2010**

I am now living fully in my body with good healthy food, comfortable clothing, warm opulent shelter and safe transportation; I am afforded freedom now from excessive toil. A Pocket Full of Wisdom **2010**

I am easily and effortlessly afforded the right balance of quality rest and fabulously fun recreation necessary to my optimal physical and emotional well-being. A Pocket Full of Wisdom **2010**

I am enjoying fascinating and fun books, lively music, splendid entertainment, gorgeous art and culture, luxurious travel, fine cuisine, and first class luxury transportation, accommodations, services and amenities. A Pocket Full of Wisdom **2010**

I always have ample time to study, listen to beautiful music and enjoy gorgeous sceneries. I love writing, reading, love and friendship, music and stunning nature; I'm afforded and live the kind of Rich life that celebrates all of this, and more! A Pocket Full of Wisdom **2010**

I lovingly appreciate Art and Culture. I go first class as I safely travel the world. I'm a Billionaire, who lives a fabulously glamorous Rich, happy and long healthy life! A Pocket Full of Wisdom **2010**

I enjoy a balanced lifestyle with appropriate rest, relaxation and play. I am now celebrating my fabulous Rich, happy and healthy life! A Pocket Full of Wisdom **2010**

I am easily and effortlessly afforded extraordinary opportunities for optimal health, safe travel and opulent observations. I safely travel with the correct traveling companion(s) who are also affluent, trustworthy, loving, loyal, intellectual, appreciative and fun-loving! A Pocket Full of Wisdom **2010**

To live fully in mind I have intellectual recreations, and I surround myself with all the objects of art and beauty I am capable of using and appreciating. A Pocket Full of Wisdom **2010**

And the two shall become one!
I am living fully in my soul, enjoying the correct love relationship (Marriage) in my life under grace and in a perfect way, with my Supreme correct arrangement. A Pocket Full of Wisdom **2010**

I am living fully in my soul, having the correct loving Marriage, family and friendships according to a Supreme endorsement and in truth. A Pocket Full of Wisdom **2010**

I am living much happiness and I'm an irresistible magnet for receiving and giving great happiness as I bestow benefits on those I love. A Pocket Full of Wisdom **2010**

It's just so fabulous being Me! I easily, healthily and happily live a full Rich life in mind, body and spirit. A Pocket Full of Wisdom **2010**

I give my attention to God and his Kingdom, for it is the noblest and most necessary of all studies. I enjoy this duty to myself, God and humanity; as I make the most of myself daily. A Pocket Full of Wisdom **2010**

I am dealing with men, women and children who are happily and easily inclined to deal with me in the manner and ways that I want to deal, rendering Rich results. A Pocket Full of Wisdom **2010**

There are no business limitations on my pathway, therefore being Rich and Happy is not dependent upon my engaging in any particular business, but upon my doing things in the correct way. A Pocket Full of Wisdom **2010**

I acquire and I'm afforded much business capital readily time after time on my pathway. So, as I receive capital my increase is easy and rapid. *A Pocket Full of Wisdom* **2010**

As I require business capital, I receive it honestly and easily; my Rich business dealings and matters are co-created with Supreme intelligence with ease, accuracy, joy and finesse! A Pocket Full of Wisdom **2010**

I'm in the correct refined business, in the proper location, doing my business in a certain Supreme way that makes me Rich! A Pocket Full of Wisdom **2010**

Prosperity channels open easily and effortlessly for me along my pathway. I am engaging in a refined elite business in the certain way that makes me extremely Rich and happy! A Pocket Full of Wisdom **2010**

The tide of opportunity sets in different directions, according to my exact needs of the whole, therefore my wealth arrives just on time! A Pocket Full of Wisdom **2010**

I am one with the "Master Class"; therefore the law of wealth works perfectly the same for me as it is for all Billionaires. A Pocket Full of Wisdom **2010**

There is more than enough inexhaustible supply for me and my family; therefore, I am now enjoying my visible inexhaustible supply. A Pocket Full of Wisdom **2010**

God is my supply and things naturally respond to my needs; therefore, I'm not without any good thing required or desired!
A Pocket Full of Wisdom **2010**

*God increases my territory!
I am continually enjoying life more; my boundaries are always extending for a fuller expression of true love, joy, optimal health, and wealth!* A Pocket Full of Wisdom **2010**

God is such a Marvelous Living Presence, always moving inherently toward more life and fuller functioning for me and mine. A Pocket Full of Wisdom **2010**

I joyfully and healthily spring into activity. The act of living produces hundreds more seeds of Prosperity! A Pocket Full of Wisdom **2010**

The life I'm living, increases. I am forever becoming Richer and Happier every day and night! A Pocket Full of Wisdom **2010**

I give every man and women for which I am in business transactions more in value than I take from them! A Pocket Full of Wisdom **2010**

There is no competition in Divine Mind. I am already Rich, so I do not need to work in a competitive way. A Pocket Full of Wisdom **2010**

I do not need to beat anybody in business because I am already Rich and I'm a winner either way! A Pocket Full of Wisdom **2010**

I am always adding to the life of the world by every business transaction I do! A Pocket Full of Wisdom **2010**

I never hesitate about asking largely; since "it's my Father's pleasure to give me the Kingdom," according to Jesus Christ. A Pocket Full of Wisdom **2010**

God works mysteriously and gracefully in me to do for his Glorification! A Pocket Full of Wisdom **2010**

I never hesitate to ask largely, since my part is to focalize and express my true hearts desires to God! A Pocket Full of Wisdom **2010**

I continually and fervently hold the whole vision of my desires; the whole picture in my mind, until what I want that is divinely for me is a part of my life! A Pocket Full of Wisdom **2010**

I live fully in my body with good food and nutrition, physical health and fitness, comfortable and lavish clothing, elegant warm and safe shelter; and with freedom from excessive toil. A Pocket Full of Wisdom **2010**

I enjoy fun recreational activities and proper rest. My energy soars since I always enjoy optimal health necessary to living a balanced lifestyle. A Pocket Full of Wisdom **2010**

God is never too late! It is unnecessary for me to ever pray repeatedly to God for the desires of my heart; God answers Divine Prayers and Promises as each one is asked, likewise they are answered just on time! A Pocket Full of Wisdom **2010**

I easily and effortlessly "pray without ceasing", always holding steadily to my vision, with the purpose to cause its creation into solid form, with tremendous faith that it is done by the Supreme for the good of all concerned! A Pocket Full of Wisdom **2010**

I am thoroughly at ease as I address Infinite Spirit in reverent prayer; and from this moment, I wholly believe and receive that the Divine delivers readily what I ask – for the good of all concerned. A Pocket Full of Wisdom **2010**

I do not need to compel God to give me good things because as certain and as timely as the Sun rises, I am certain I am not without every good thing! A Pocket Full of Wisdom **2010**

I am Rich and happy by simply using will power upon myself, holding course with the Mastermind with love, faith and good purpose. I exercise my Supreme will "power" to achieve great success! A Pocket Full of Wisdom **2010**

I put poverty or any idea of struggle or loss behind me; I make "Good" by being Rich, which is the best, most honorable and divine way for me to help myself! Likewise, I richly and blissfully advance helping becoming men, women and children, and the poor. A Pocket Full of Wisdom **2010**

I help the becoming men, women and children and the poor by being "Inspiring"; I always demonstrate how easily and rapidly they can be Rich; I prove it by demonstration, being Rich myself! A Pocket Full of Wisdom **2010**

I reverently inspire large masses of people, constantly increasing my own Wealth and Happiness by paving the way and teaching "Rich Proclamations" of how to become Rich also; for it is the best I can do for my fellowman. A Pocket Full of Wisdom **2010**

I spread "Rich Proclamations" of the "Good" news and Supreme Power is eminent.

God creates a Mighty and Victorious Safe pathway for me and many thousands that want to come along; I am one who is "Rich"! A Pocket Full of Wisdom **2010**

Christ lives! "let the dead bury their dead," and "I dissolve poverty and all things that pertain to poverty; all past troubles of financial nature are completely dissolved now under Supreme and in a proper way! A Pocket Full of Wisdom **2010**

I am a Legacy of Love and I'm Rich!

I do not think of poverty at all, only wealth now! I richly and worthily contribute to my Community and the World so I easily and effectually make a real difference! A Pocket Full of Wisdom **2010**

There is only one power for me, and that is of the Marvelous Power of God! A Pocket Full of Wisdom **2010**

The world and I am with God; it is a Marvelous becoming! A Pocket Full of Wisdom **2010**

My noblest aim is being Rich; I am experiencing the fullest expression of life, for it includes everything else! A Pocket Full of Wisdom **2010**

I see the Truth of my Great One Life ever moving forward toward fuller expression and more complete happiness! A Pocket Full of Wisdom **2010**

My most certain and best contribution and purpose in my life to this world is to make the most of myself. This includes being healthy, happy and Rich; for then I am also the giver and the gift unto others in this World. A Pocket Full of Wisdom **2010**

I am poised and my words are established correctly with poise! I genuinely give a smile to the stranger and reverently inspire the World with words of Wisdom! A Pocket Full of Wisdom **2010**

Infinite Spirit goes before me, and divinely inspires me as I make the Best of myself and likewise inspire others! A Pocket Full of Wisdom **2010**

Together with God, I am Co-creator in this vast Universe! Therefore, the propelling power of the Supreme Spirit, leads me from everlasting-to-everlasting Riches! A Pocket Full of Wisdom **2010**

God prepares a Victorious way for me; in every transaction I am led in a certain way that my storehouse of lavish treasures is poured upon me; I receive it with gratitude, love and understanding! A Pocket Full of Wisdom **2010**

I easily and effortlessly hold onto the purpose to get what I want; and in realizing with faith and gratitude that I do get what I want for the good of all concerned! A Pocket Full of Wisdom **2010**

In a creative nature I rightly give to my fellowman; as I arrange my own business affairs to be prepared as I rightly receive what I want as it reaches me! A Pocket Full of Wisdom **2010**

I set the creative forces of the Powerful Universe into positive effect; now I have more abundant and joyful life and affluence directed to me! A Pocket Full of Wisdom **2010**

I act now in love under Supreme Influence using my natural capabilities, talents and abilities to co-create a marvelous, healthy, happy Rich life for myself! A Pocket Full of Wisdom **2010**

I am actively competent each day, giving the most of myself leaving no good stone unturned. A Pocket Full of Wisdom **2010**

I act now in Love under Supreme Influence using my natural capabilities, talents and abilities to co-create a marvelous, healthy, happy Rich life for myself! A Pocket Full of Wisdom **2010**

I am an advancing Rich person in mind, body and spirit, actively living today in absolute Faith that I am Rich. Today, I move forward with a powerful Rich purpose in Supreme ways! A Pocket Full of Wisdom **2010**

Better for me, and better for others that I am Rich. The Richer for me now, the better! I now sow the seeds and proclaim that my wealth and eternal increase pours out upon me in a waterfall of Poise and Prosperity!

I now sow the seeds and proclaim that my wealth and eternal increase pours out upon me in a waterfall of Poise and Prosperity!

Better for me, and better for others that I am Rich. The Richer for me now, the better!

Better for me, and better for others that I am Rich. The Richer for me now, the better! A Pocket Full of Wisdom **2010**

I cast away any troubles and sink them
into the depths of the sea;
Now my treasure is found here in me! A
Pocket Full of Wisdom **2010**

I am Safe, I am Home; God is Here; I'm not alone! A Pocket Full of Wisdom **2010**

I am a citizen of the Kingdom of Heaven; therefore everything that is for me in Heaven is also for me here on Earth!
A Pocket Full of Wisdom **2010**

Any and all obstructions no matter how great, dissipate as I approach it; Or else a way over, though, or around it easily and miraculously appears and I am Victorious in Christ! A Pocket Full of Wisdom **2010**

My Love and Joy is increased, pressed down and multiplied. I obey Universal Laws; I am established and eternally Rich! A Pocket Full of Wisdom **2010**

I give no anxious thought to possible disasters, obstacles, panics, or adverse conditions in my life, and I am extremely confident that if presented with any difficulty, I'm given the ease and courage to arise triumphantly! A Pocket Full of Wisdom **2010**

I speak of my own personal and business affairs and anything else in the most encouraging and inspiring ways! A Pocket Full of Wisdom **2010**

Christ is with me and I am free; nothing therefore bothers me! A Pocket Full of Wisdom **2010**

I am confident and poised; I'm enough for me and thee! I am God's child and I go free! A Pocket Full of Wisdom **2010**

I honor and respect Universal Law; I worthily adhere to the prevailing Supreme power of spoken words, thoughts, or deeds, especially the Law of Attraction. A Pocket Full of Wisdom **2010**

I am far above fear or doubt; I create absolutely everything I want, and need. Rejoice! Times are always straightforward and thereby Rich for me! A Pocket Full of Wisdom **2010**

Rejoice! My everlasting faith and love does not toil to advance, become and grow! With pleasure, I delight in the truth that this is so! A Pocket Full of Wisdom **2010**

I am never met with defeat! Any seeming failure works out correctly for me as I keep the faith, hold to my vision, give gratitude, and seize Liberty and Wealth from everlasting-to-everlasting! A Pocket Full of Wisdom **2010**

I wholly harvest and develop all the talent that is within me to do the kind of work I love in fabulous ways; with increasingly Rich magnificent pay! A Pocket Full of Wisdom **2010**

Christ lives! My true life story is one of Glory! A Pocket Full of Wisdom **2010**

My life has an extraordinary Divine Purpose; so I live it with the utmost honor and reverence to the Infinite Spirit of Creation! A Pocket Full of Wisdom **2010**

I am adorned in full harmony by Supreme Power; I entertain a lively and sincere appreciation for the blessings bestowed upon me by the living loving God Almighty. A Pocket Full of Wisdom **2010**

Each transaction in my life creates more positive life; I hold to the advancing thoughts that the impression of increase is made in me; likewise, I effectively and concisely communicate this to all with whom I deal. A Pocket Full of Wisdom **2010**

I am Rich and Happy! Behold, I am celebrating Prosperity life in my sound and balanced mind, body and spirit! A Pocket Full of Wisdom **2010**

I am free and unhampered to use of every good thing that is required for me to be abundantly happy and rich to its fullest mental, spiritual, and physical enfoldment. A Pocket Full of Wisdom **2010**

I'm capable of using and enjoying more in my life, so nature and Supreme Authority contributes to the power, elegance, beauty, and fullness of my life! A Pocket Full of Wisdom **2010**

I am fully capable, talented, and confident at just the "Ripe Time" to be all that I can be according to God's Divine Plan.
A Pocket Full of Wisdom **2010**

I enjoy great true love all of my days and nights; love is expressed in optimal health, joy, peace, faith, hope and love. I give and receive "Good Love" easily and effortlessly under Supreme Power with poise! A Pocket Full of Wisdom **2010**

I easily and effortlessly Co-create with the Universal Laws as I cultivate my talents and natural abilities to be Rich and Abundantly Happy! A Pocket Full of Wisdom **2010**

Everything and anyone I need or require for my being happy, healthy and rich is manifested along my pathway. I always engage in the correct business transactions yielding extraordinary success and prosperity!
A Pocket Full of Wisdom **2010**

As certain as the Sun rises in the East and sets in the West; as certain as there is North and South – From every direction I receive the sweet wind of Prosperity, Love and Joy season-after-season, year-after-year! A Pocket Full of Wisdom **2010**

I Co-create words of the Spirit that heal. I am an Eternal Legacy of Love and Good Tidings. My good words and deeds herewith God shall never return void as they accomplish great and marvelous outcomes throughout the Earth.

A Pocket Full of Wisdom **2010**

Today, opportunity is open, so the correct Doors of Success welcome me as I enter into my correct professional and personal Endeavors of Successes! A Pocket Full of Wisdom **2010**

I effortlessly, respectfully, and wisely come and go through the correct Doors of Success with a Rich outcome of financial freedom, ease, poise, and grace! A Pocket Full of Wisdom **2010**

What is not eventually or ever meant for me by the Supreme Authority dissolves along my path before I approach. Angels guide and protect me along my pathway. A Pocket Full of Wisdom **2010**

What relationships are not eventually or ever for me dissolve along my path before I approach. Behold! What is for me I am victorious to achieve and receive and I cannot ever lose what is rightfully mine to keep! A Pocket Full of Wisdom **2010**

What relationships are not eventually or ever for me dissolve along my path before I approach. Behold! What is for me I am victorious to achieve and receive and I cannot ever loose what is rightfully mine to keep and love the most! A Pocket Full of Wisdom **2010**

Now I lay me down to sleep, what's mine is mine; I get to keep. Think Happy and Rich each night and day. My Joys, Spirit shall never take away!
A Pocket Full of Wisdom **2010**

What I'm meant to keep that is mine I keep and what is not for me dissolves easily and effortlessly before approach! A Pocket Full of Wisdom **2010**

Only the best, loving, safest and correct people, things and circumstances are for me and near me under Supreme Grace and in the most ideal ways! A Pocket Full of Wisdom **2010**

All positive appearances are the God Power at work in my life; so nothing else can enter in but what is of good and worthy report under Supreme Grace and in the most ideal ways! A Pocket Full of Wisdom **2010**

There is only God Power in my life now! Today, I'm thinking and becoming... advancing to Optimal Health, Wealth, Love, Powerful Light Energy and Joy! A Pocket Full of Wisdom **2010**

I enjoy fun-filled relationships and I foster great friendships, love and peace to all whom I meet. A Pocket Full of Wisdom
2010

Hark! I experience the same good dealing and good tidings in return for the goodness that I give; likewise, I am receiving in exceptionally good measure! A Pocket Full of Wisdom **2010**

I do not take things personally since I know that God has the power to heal all things great and small; Indeed it's true, the good God does it All! A Pocket Full of Wisdom **2010**

*I am unconcerned of any fear on my way;
The Supreme Being is here to stay.* A
Pocket Full of Wisdom **2010**

No worries; No anxious thoughts in me; God is my Serenity! A Pocket Full of Wisdom **2010**

Behold! I have no fear!
What never happened in the Kingdom,
likewise never happens here. A Pocket Full of
Wisdom **2010**

I'm unconcerned with the appearances of things as the Lions lay down gracefully and peacefully with the Lambs on my pathway! A Pocket Full of Wisdom **2010**

I release damaged things and circumstances from my past and go free in the present with true love, forgiveness and understanding. A Pocket Full of Wisdom **2010**

I am healed by the Supreme One; all worn out things are finished; I'm new, advancing, and I am ceaselessly Rich, Healthy, and Happy! A Pocket Full of Wisdom **2010**

I act according to raison d'être, desiring from God what's good for me! A Pocket Full of Wisdom **2010**

I act correctly, according to faith and reason; I always promote only good, not only for me but also for others. A Pocket Full of Wisdom **2010**

My life pleasures arise from creating adequate ideas! I correctly develop these first-rate ideas with Infinite Spirit. A Pocket Full of Wisdom **2010**

Infinite Intelligence in my sound mind, body and spirit adequately expresses an essence of God. A Pocket Full of Wisdom **2010**

I am Virtuous, thereby enjoying adequate Spiritual knowledge and perception. A Pocket Full of Wisdom **2010**

I correctly act according to faith and Supreme Truth. I'm guided by Heavenly Angels abounding true love and good-will; not by any fear or hatred. A Pocket Full of Wisdom **2010**

The better I control my emotions; the better I understand God.
The better I am. *A Pocket Full of Wisdom* **2010**

I now and continually enjoy pleasure in the contemplation of God's perfections, as is the way of genuine 'pure love,' which I actively give gratification for my delight and the happiness of my beloved. A Pocket Full of Wisdom **2010**

I am a Virtuous being devoting my energies to everything which is harmonious according to the presumptive or antecedent will of God. A Pocket Full of Wisdom

2010

I am satisfied and content in my soul what my God truly brings to pass for me, His Marvelous Secrets unfolding and astonishing. A Pocket Full of Wisdom **2010**

God's power and gifts to me exceed all my desires and astound even the wisest and richest men! A Pocket Full of Wisdom **2010**

The Creator of all, and the most efficient cause of my being, is my God; my Master and final cause is the aim of my will ... which can alone, afford all of my happiness. A Pocket Full of Wisdom **2010**

I am more than just Lucky, Or, Rich! I am constant, precise and I infuse the essence of God. A Pocket Full of Wisdom **2010**

I Co-create with the Infinite Spirit with a kind of eloquence and power that accomplishes great and marvelous workings!
A Pocket Full of Wisdom **2010**

I connect with the Divine that demonstrates Powerful Wealth-building opportunities to me. I focus and do what is good, what is lovely, and what is true and upright.

Behold my path is made straight, the roads easily traveled, and the gates of Richness, my inheritance is wide open! A Pocket Full of Wisdom **2010**

I am a necessity in spirit and flesh, manifesting God itself, always glorifying, advancing and becoming! A Pocket Full of Wisdom **2010**

I celebrate life, especially nature, love, light, what is virtuous and of Spiritual Truth. A Pocket Full of Wisdom **2010**

Infinite Spirit goes ahead of me and with a Marvelous ease, offering up all its kingdoms to me which I may mould into what is valuable. A Pocket Full of Wisdom **2010**

Behold! .... I have Infinite access to the entire mind of the Creator. A Pocket Full of Wisdom **2010**

Nothing can become an object for me. Everything moves seamlessly with ease along my pathway. A Pocket Full of Wisdom **2010**

Space and time work perfectly for me because God is always precisely on time! A Pocket Full of Wisdom **2010**

I am receiving the correct nourishment for my optimal internal and external health and also in my physical and spiritual body A Pocket Full of Wisdom **2010**

My health is extraordinary; Infinite Spirit nourishes my every cell and they are illuminated with Supreme light. A Pocket Full of Wisdom **2010**

I am eternally grateful for my extraordinary health, eternal happiness, permanent love, and infinite joy! A Pocket Full of Wisdom **2010**

I am the Supreme's eyes, ears, and voice; and I further to complete a Divine plan formed in me. A Pocket Full of Wisdom **2010**

I live an increasingly richly expressive life; so naturally, I receive the gifts of the Kingdom easily here on Earth. A Pocket Full of Wisdom **2010**

I am loving, harmonious and happy; therefore I have perfect well-balanced health. A Pocket Full of Wisdom **2010**

I live the unique extraordinary life that only I can live according to the Supreme, and I am infinitely happy and Rich as I do so! A Pocket Full of Wisdom **2010**

What is not of the Divine Principle Plan cannot be; for there is only "One God Power" in me! A Pocket Full of Wisdom **2010**

I am seamlessly connected to all of the correct persons, things and circumstances that excel me to be my absolute best and to live a Divine existence of good tidings now! A Pocket Full of Wisdom **2010**

Ask, Seek, Knock!
I ask God humbly, for the things that
I want.
I seek God in All matters, big and
small.
I knock at the door of Heaven and
The Good Lord answers me. A Pocket
Full of Wisdom **2010**

I am unconcerned with the darkness; only God Power and Infinite Light exist for me! A Pocket Full of Wisdom **2010**

I am anxious for nothing; I trust God and everything goes accordingly. A Pocket Full of Wisdom **2010**

I celebrate Joy everyday and I reverently and happily do what must be done for this day. A Pocket Full of Wisdom **2010**

I dance and leap for joy as I receive money, checks, gifts and fabulous Rich surprises mysteriously appear before my eyes, meant only for me! A Pocket Full of Wisdom **2010**

I am afforded all of the luxurious and opulent gifts and first fruits of the Infinite Spirit and I gloriously praise and celebrate receiving Supreme Goods and Services in my Rich life! A Pocket Full of Wisdom **2010**

Glorious ways and glorious days are mine forever and a day! A Pocket Full of Wisdom
2010

My heart is gloriously happy for the goodness and majestic ways of our perfect God! A Pocket Full of Wisdom **2010**

.

I am unconcerned with the things that aren't mine; I trust explicitly the Divine!
A Pocket Full of Wisdom **2010**

My truth is sealed in the Spirit of God; Jesus Christ is the worthy one who I adore, the "Only One!" A Pocket Full of Wisdom **2010**

Regards, the past is gone! I forgive the rest; I receive the Best now in mutual love and understanding! A Pocket Full of Wisdom **2010**

I am present and much alive!
Today, I am a gift; a life. A Pocket Full
of Wisdom **2010**

Today and Tomorrow I am here to glorify Infinite Spirit and powerfully manifest Spirit Love throughout the Earth. My Heavenly Richness reaches Earth and creates Wealth for me out of mysterious places and spaces of the Universe. A Pocket Full of Wisdom **2010**

I am growing and increasing in Wisdom. I listen more, talk less and speak the truth. A Pocket Full of Wisdom **2010**

I say the things of Infinite Spirit and hold my tongue for that which is not love and truth. A Pocket Full of Wisdom **2010**

I am wise in my dealings with others. All men, women and children know God quite simply for knowing me! A Pocket Full of Wisdom **2010**

God is perfect in all ways! So, there is no imperfection for me. It is only perfection perceiving yet imperfect ideas. A Pocket Full of Wisdom **2010**

I am likened as the fresh morning bloom, opening with ease and beauty – just as I am, never too late, never too soon! A Pocket Full of Wisdom **2010**

The sun is effortless to rise; as such I rise above circumstances and appearances that are not becoming; or, of good and worthy account. *A Pocket Full of Wisdom* **2010**

I smile fluently genuine and true; a smile is easier than a frown and takes less effort too! So, this is what I do! I Smile for you! A Pocket Full of Wisdom **2010**

I am self-assuredly poised; my posture and gate is physically powerful as I go forth with eloquence and proper beauty! A Pocket Full of Wisdom **2010**

I am well esteemed and sought by the highest, most honorable and respectable individuals for my loving and supreme intellect, and my fun-loving personality! A Pocket Full of Wisdom **2010**

I give from the heart. I make Good life-long friendships easily; Likewise, I also receive the best treatments and adornments for my gracious hospitality! A Pocket Full of Wisdom **2010**

I receive astonishing amounts and figures of currency, money, checks, capital, resources, investments, and assets to do what is good and of worthy report to the Supreme! A Pocket Full of Wisdom **2010**

I have good and plenty! So, now I'm significantly afforded to happily adorn others with my warmth and giving nature and outstanding hospitality! A Pocket Full of Wisdom **2010**

I go to the most extraordinary and lavish destinations. All of my travel is lovely, peaceful, and I move along easily on my journey, arriving safely and happily to my easily afforded aim. A Pocket Full of Wisdom **2010**

Marvelous and opulent gifts and surprises are provided to me here on Earth poured out in lavish arrangements from the Kingdom. A Pocket Full of Wisdom **2010**

I am safe, balanced and at home in my own physical, emotional and spiritual mind, body and spirit! A Pocket Full of Wisdom **2010**

I have exhilarating work in a supernatural way; I give delightful service for miraculous pay! A Pocket Full of Wisdom **2010**

My Prosperity and Joy is unrelenting; I have a sense of well-being and internal peace that surpasses all of my potential! A Pocket Full of Wisdom **2010**

Hark, I hear with clarity my soulful purpose from Infinite Wisdom; the Almighty Supreme gives me clarity beyond recognition to do incredibly Rich things! A Pocket Full of Wisdom **2010**

Hark! I hear the clear sound of peace!
A Pocket Full of Wisdom **2010**

Behold, only the best of people, things and circumstances; or, best intentions are provided to me now! A Pocket Full of Wisdom **2010**

My Guardian Angels soar. I love and thank my Angels who bravely, courageously love and protect me and mine. Infinite Spirit gives Angel orders and my Angels most certainly excel victoriously! A Pocket Full of Wisdom **2010**

Behold, I proclaim only the highest and richest possibilities to shine upon me, over and under my foot. My feet are established and are Holy and upright in character! A Pocket Full of Wisdom **2010**

I am like the graceful gazelle, swiftly motivated with beauty and grace! A Pocket Full of Wisdom **2010**

My temperament is sophisticated, lovely and affectionate; my yoke is easy! A Pocket Full of Wisdom **2010**

My intelligence and wit is as crafty and cunning as the Fox. I can "outfox" any Good thing out of a box! A Pocket Full of Wisdom **2010**

I am adorable, playful and fun-loving with all of the charm, sophistication and thrill of the playful Fox! A Pocket Full of Wisdom **2010**

I am happy to be charitable with my Riches. I affordably tithe with great tidings and joy no less than 10 percent to the Poor with the first fruits of my Richness and Prosperity! A Pocket Full of Wisdom **2010**

I'm exactly the right and correct healthy Rich person for my companion and likewise. My companion has found me and we are divinely joined together in love and understanding by Infinite Spirit. A Pocket Full of Wisdom **2010**

My Children are safe, healthy and happy – living under Infinite Spirit's protection and law and nothing can change the perfect Love of God in me for my Children; and vice versa. A Pocket Full of Wisdom **2010**

From generation to generation my Kingdom come, my will be done and shall be an inheritance to the youth who continue on this Earth when I arrive in Heaven! A Pocket Full of Wisdom **2010**

I am a Legacy of Love for the Universal Men, Women and Children. I am an inspiration, motivational truth in the light of God's Power! A Pocket Full of Wisdom **2010**

My words and thoughts are careful and well chosen to continually align more readily with Infinite Spirit. *A Pocket Full of Wisdom* **2010**

My thoughts and actions are aligned with a careful Supreme guided consciousness to do what is upright, worthy, and of good report! A Pocket Full of Wisdom **2010**

God is so worthy!
God is the One Power, Supreme Giver, and the Gift who righteously and mightily answers me; just as I am! A Pocket Full of Wisdom **2010**

I receive astonishing amounts and figures of currency, money, checks, capital, resources, investments, assets to do what is good and of worthy report to the Supreme! A Pocket Full of Wisdom **2010**

All matters, people, circumstances or things that are not useful or helpful in my life are dissolved and replaced with valuable and obliging ventures and adventures! A Pocket Full of Wisdom **2010**

The seed is sown, the tree is planted, its roots are strong, justified, and thriving... I am like a tree by the living waters drinking the fountain of youth and the way of life, Lord Jesus. A Pocket Full of Wisdom **2010**

Behold, I aspire to my unique natural talents and capabilities and I shine free to be me. A Pocket Full of Wisdom **2010**

Unswerving tides wash and carry away any troubles or wrong appearances. Whisked away and never to be; yeah, cast into the depths of the deep blue sea! A Pocket Full of Wisdom **2010**

Infinite Spirit says "Yes" to the Divine Plan and they are made manifest in me now in marvelous ways! A Pocket Full of Wisdom **2010**

I now possess the drive and ambition to achieve my wildest dreams and more; I have come out of the jungle and arrived at Paradise! A Pocket Full of Wisdom **2010**

All of my needs are infinitely managed and provided by the Kingdom, I am feeling achievement, good health and wealth! A Pocket Full of Wisdom **2010**

It's time to celebrate because now, I am achieving and receiving! A Pocket Full of Wisdom **2010**

What rings true to bring honest riches divinely to others rings true for me too! The Prosperity Bell is sounding and its resonance is crystal clear, my prosperity appointed time is here! A Pocket Full of Wisdom **2010**

Now is my appointed time of Wealth, Optimal Health, Love, Joy, and Peace! I am like a Rare and Precious Diamond of Richness sparkling, shimmering in the light. A Pocket Full of Wisdom **2010**

Now is my appointed time of Wealth, I am the ripe bloom! My fragrance of success shines throughout the world; the morning dew quenches! The sweetness of love and gratitude reaches from Heaven to Earth.

A Pocket Full of Wisdom **2010**

Ripe as a berry, seen by a bird soaring across the land, my mind, soul and body is nourished richly by God's sacred and Holy hands! A Pocket Full of Wisdom **2010**

I am anxious for nothing on the highways and byways of life. All of the traffic goes smoothly, peacefully, safely and everything flows and goes agreeably on my journey! A Pocket Full of Wisdom **2010**

All my adventures and travels in life are well routed, easily afforded, luxurious and safe for me and thee; who go along my journey. A Pocket Full of Wisdom **2010**

All of my travels along my journey coming to and fro, coming out and going in are safe, peaceful, and everything flows richly and goes agreeably for me and also for all who journey along with me! A Pocket Full of Wisdom **2010**

I travel to Rich exciting and opulent destinations. I celebrate life on the road of success and give reverence on these journeys to Infinite Spirit for such marvelous beauty, nature, quality service, ease and personal safety for myself and my traveling companion(s). A Pocket Full of Wisdom **2010**

God's timing is above reproach! The One and Only Power who is the Immaculate Spirit of God is "Just on Time"! Hence, I honor and respect the time of others with Poise and always aim to arrive, a few minutes early or just on time! A Pocket Full of Wisdom **2010**

I choose my esteemed friends and colleagues ever so wisely according to the prodding of the Infinite Spirit. I pay attention to these promptings so that any apparent obstacle, threat or visible enemy or adversary power is immediately dissolved under Supreme protection for me. A Pocket Full of Wisdom **2010**

I have now in my possession and thereby use the Golden Key of Success that unlocks extraordinary wealth, health and happiness for me. A Pocket Full of Wisdom
2010

I have now in my possession and thereby use the Golden Key of Success, which has astonishing Infinite Powers and it has a clearly unlocked unobstructed wealthy passages, so I now receive my hearts desires! *A Pocket Full of Wisdom* **2010**

Infinite Spirit proclaims that I am already Rich! Therefore, I am now experiencing and enjoying an extraordinary measure of wealth being poured out in waterfalls of Richness, Joy and Love, here on Earth as it is in Heaven. A Pocket Full of Wisdom **2010**

My soul is at peace! Infinite Spirit is the One and Only Power worthy to open the seal. Heavenly hosts praise and glorify as I daily live for this One Power who is, God – This is where my treasure is. A Pocket Full of Wisdom **2010**

My infinite blessings flow where love goes. Coming in and going out, Love flows easily and effortlessly. My great love is given and great love is reciprocated with Supreme poise and perfection! A Pocket Full of Wisdom **2010**

My Spirit light shines brightly; I'm a dawning star and I am wonderfully made uprightly! A Pocket Full of Wisdom **2010**

As certain as the sun rises and sets, Supreme is from everlasting-to-everlasting and I too! God lives in me and you. A Pocket Full of Wisdom **2010**

As fluidly as the cloud formations in the sky take shape, my Wealth is fashioned never too late! A Pocket Full of Wisdom **2010**

My mind is sharp with wellness, clarity, intelligence, wisdom and peace. Peace every day and never the least! A Pocket Full of Wisdom **2010**

I am an enticement for perpetual increase, optimal health, prosperity, richness, happiness and love; time after time! A Pocket Full of Wisdom **2010**

My spirit and spiritual energy is astounding, vibrant and wholesome! A Pocket Full of Wisdom **2010**

Today, I am young-looking, young at heart, optimally healthy, happy, loving, fun-loving, vibrant and alive for such a time as this! A Pocket Full of Wisdom **2010**

Today, my physical and emotional health is paramount and I enjoy optimal health, perpetual Riches and happiness day upon day, year upon year; time after time! A Pocket Full of Wisdom **2010**

Wherever I am going, Infinite Spirit is my compass; I set appropriate course and arrive precisely where I'm to be; Spirit never too late for me! A Pocket Full of Wisdom **2010**

I ask and receive because I believe,
Infinite Power I thank Thee! A
Pocket Full of Wisdom **2010**

I seek and receive answers because I believe; Infinite Power does it for me! A Pocket Full of Wisdom **2010**

*I knock at the door of Heaven and
Christ I see; Holy Spirit answers me!*
A Pocket Full of Wisdom **2010**

I foster and enjoy amazing friendships in understanding and love; I thank thee God above! A Pocket Full of Wisdom **2010**

.

Well into my Golden Years, I am a pinnacle of extraordinary health and fitness and perpetual Richness. I live a Joy-filled existence as my body ages ever so gently with ease. A Pocket Full of Wisdom **2010**

My Golden Years are filled with Joy-filled living, loving, and happiness. My healthy golden years shall serve my soul well and do what is good and of worthy report! A Pocket Full of Wisdom **2010**

Now and into my Golden Years, I am blessed and living a legacy of love, prosperity, and good health that I enjoy from generation to generation to generation!
A Pocket Full of Wisdom **2010**

I adapt to the changes on Earth as easily and effortlessly as it is in Heaven. A Pocket Full of Wisdom **2010**

I live a happy Rich life with an unshakeable faith! A Pocket Full of Wisdom
2010

I always adapt to the ever changing world around me with ease; I am a wise and becoming character with immense integrity!
A Pocket Full of Wisdom **2010**

I am flexible and poised as I listen and hear my fellow man's points of view as I maintain and conclude astute decisions. A Pocket Full of Wisdom **2010**

I am not easily confused, I listen and hear my fellow man and reach an incisive and meaningful conclusion for the good of all concerned. A Pocket Full of Wisdom **2010**

I am reasonable and understood, I listen and hear my fellow man and reach an incisive and meaningful conclusion for the good of all concerned. A Pocket Full of Wisdom **2010**

I express my thoughts and ideas with forward thinking clear and decisive implementation; therefore I'm understood easily and effortlessly in my Personal and Business dealings. A Pocket Full of Wisdom **2010**

I live a fair, poised, well groomed and well-spoken lifestyle. Behold, I'm harmonious in my personal and business dealings, circumstances or consequences! A Pocket Full of Wisdom **2010**

I am poised, proper, well groomed, promoted and well-favored in my dealings with others, therefore other's deal with me in a certain way that is poised and correct. A Pocket Full of Wisdom **2010**

I am well sought, well thought, and well promoted in my dealings and treatments of others and likewise I enjoy extraordinary Riches and Happiness! A Pocket Full of Wisdom **2010**

I am well spiritually well-established: I effectively aim to adhere to Supreme universal principles that are most legitimate, holy and acceptable in their applicability, intellectual and financial stature, translation, and philosophical and/or spiritual views. A Pocket Full of Wisdom **2010**

I'm motivated today to do the most and best efficient Rich efforts, seeking a fuller expression of Infinite Spirit in all of my personal and business dealings. A Pocket Full of Wisdom **2010**

My home is a peaceful, prosperous, safe and harmonious sanctuary of love! A Pocket Full of Wisdom **2010**

Happiness and love abides in my happy home and all who enter into it enjoy the finest hospitality provided by the most gracious host of the most! A Pocket Full of Wisdom **2010**

I am tireless and energetic and my energy is magnetic and enticing! A Pocket Full of Wisdom **2010**

I am industrious, bold, confident and beautiful, unique in just the right way: mind, body and spirit by God! A Pocket Full of Wisdom **2010**

My luminous ideas manifest easily and I am Rich; Money and checks flow to me without a hitch! A Pocket Full of Wisdom **2010**

As bars of gold shimmer and shine, eternal wealth and good health and good tidings are mine! A Pocket Full of Wisdom *2010*

As the salty sea sparkles and shines; the treasure found, is mine! A Pocket Full of Wisdom **2010**

Whatever is required or made complete; it is finished so I don't compete! A Pocket Full of Wisdom **2010**

I discover new, easy and exciting methods to accomplish my goals and ambitions with ease and gratification! A Pocket Full of Wisdom **2010**

I am forgiven and I am free; God's glorified and I thank Thee! A Pocket Full of Wisdom **2010**

There are no missing ideas in Spirit; therefore, Divine ideas are formed in my mind and arrive as perpetual Riches for me, just on time! A Pocket Full of Wisdom **2010**

I act in faith as planned by Infinite Spirit from the beginning, and now, I am winning! A Pocket Full of Wisdom **2010**

I deliver perfect goods and services to the best of my ability with the guidance from the Supreme! A Pocket Full of Wisdom **2010**

I act and behave in all honesty with such words and actions of sincerity! A Pocket Full of Wisdom **2010**

It is virtuous for me to act faithfully and my true virtue is my Love for God! A Pocket Full of Wisdom **2010**

I seek the knowledge of good and truth in all matters! Therefore, much good arises from my adequate ideas, especially ideas that adequately refer to God. A Pocket Full of Wisdom **2010**

In my life as cause is given, the effect that follows is very good and profitable for me! A Pocket Full of Wisdom **2010**

I am energetic, vibrant and motivated to do well, which states that my definite course of action inevitably brings about Victory! A Pocket Full of Wisdom **2010**

I am motivated from within with intuition, perception, or conception to act and/or behave according to exemplary character. A Pocket Full of Wisdom **2010**

I seek the knowledge of good and truth; therefore, much good arises from my adequate ideas, especially ideas that adequately refer to God. A Pocket Full of Wisdom **2010**

My mind is now open to Nature's beautiful influence and a kindred impression is upon me! A Pocket Full of Wisdom **2010**

In my life as cause is given, the effect that follows is very good and perpetually prosperous! A Pocket Full of Wisdom **2010**

I am energetic, vibrant and motivated to do well, which states that my definite course of action inevitably brings about Victory! A Pocket Full of Wisdom **2010**

I am motivated from within with intuition, perception, or conception to act and/or behave according to exemplary character. A Pocket Full of Wisdom **2010**

My reverence with Heaven and Earth is a part of my daily provisions. A Pocket Full of Wisdom **2010**

I seize the moment with Love and Joy as each second, minute, hour and season yields its tribute of delight; Oh, Holy are you God of Power, God of Light. A Pocket Full of Wisdom **2010**

Butterflies swoop down from the skies to carry our burdens away; they bring forth their delight, their lovely wings in flight, and I never shall dismay! A Pocket Full of Wisdom **2010**

*Precious blooms in the garden of life shine
your smiles upon thee! Rays of light
through the cedar trees; Angels in flight and
Spirit in me!* A Pocket Full of Wisdom
2010

A tiny seed was planted; then from the north, south, east, and west the wind and the rain came. Heavenly blooms unfold amidst the morning dew; Behold, Paradise is dawning in my Garden of Life. Somehow, I always knew! A Pocket Full of Wisdom **2010**

Nature affords me such natural Riches of its dowry and estate; Infinite Spirit of God, never too late! A Pocket Full of Wisdom **2010**

I'm Victorious now, I give my best; God does all the rest! A Pocket Full of Wisdom **2010**

I am an eternally youthful, fun-loving and an unshakeable Spirit from everlasting-to-everlasting! A Pocket Full of Wisdom **2010**

I am a compass I know Thy ways through the winds, the swells, and the storms; I am the North! A Pocket Full of Wisdom **2010**

I am unconcerned with the folly or appearances of others; Instead, I focus distinctly and honestly on my own affairs and resolve to be Rich, Healthy and Happy! A Pocket Full of Wisdom **2010**

I am eagerly and easily understood by others. I state my objective and assert my character and well-being to achieve the finest rewards and wealth! A Pocket Full of Wisdom **2010**

I am unconcerned with the folly and appearances of others; instead, I focus distinctly and honestly on my own affairs and resolve to be Rich, Happy and Optimally Healthy! A Pocket Full of Wisdom **2010**

I am eagerly and easily understood by others as I state my objective and assert my character and well-being to achieve the finest rewards and wealth! A Pocket Full of Wisdom **2010**

Rich is as Rich says; likewise, I am well-spoken, deliver words clearly, precisely and talk uprightly. A Pocket Full of Wisdom
2010

Rich is as Rich does; likewise, I am well-mannered, well-behaved, precise, accurate, trustworthy, loving and loyal. I act precisely and walk uprightly. A Pocket Full of Wisdom **2010**

There is no loss or poverty in Divine mind! I can only be Rich. A Pocket Full of Wisdom **2010**

There is no anxiousness, hate, or fear in Divine mind! I am Victorious! A Pocket Full of Wisdom **2010**

There is only beauty to see; appearances are only perceptions. God's truth sets me free! A Pocket Full of Wisdom **2010**

I pay to the order of "Me": Five-million and 00/100 dollars, multiplied by three!

Now, it is complete. A Pocket Full of Wisdom **2010**

The cotton cloth and threads are forming out of the formless substance; colored checks, blue and green paper notes, are being manufactured, and gold is being mined, vaulted, and circulated especially for me! A Pocket Full of Wisdom **2010**

Millions multiplied times seven. Royalty checks written out to me, thank God in Heaven! A Pocket Full of Wisdom **2010**

There is no opposition in Divine mind. From this time forth, my mind is on course and I manifest now tremendous wealth, optimal health and fitness, and true love. A Pocket Full of Wisdom **2010**

There is no opposition in Divine mind. From this time forth, my mind is on course and nothing can interfere in my Rich blessings bestowed by Infinite Spirit. A Pocket Full of Wisdom **2010**

There is no opposition to the Supreme Rich plan for my life! Nothing can rob me from my Joy! My Joy is full and I'm Rich beyond my wildest imagination. A Pocket Full of Wisdom **2010**

From this time forth, there is nothing to oppose my God Designed marvelous Rich and Happy life! A Pocket Full of Wisdom **2010**

I live a fabulously Happy and Rich Life now! A Pocket Full of Wisdom **2010**

From this time forth, what I need to know shall be written, told, sealed and delivered safely with ease and I garner the rewards of knowledge. A Pocket Full of Wisdom **2010**

From this time forth, what I need to know shall be written, told, sealed and delivered safely with ease and I garner the rewards of a Prosperity Purposeful Life!

A Pocket Full of Wisdom **2010**

Bountiful blessings and a superfluity of good and plenty are bestowed to me by Supreme Power! A Pocket Full of Wisdom **2010**

I am a non-resistant vessel that the Supreme works through, and his Divine Plans are established in me now and come into being in miraculous and wonderful ways! A Pocket Full of Wisdom **2010**

I am obedient, humble, and divinely inspired. Supreme power directs my paths and shows me just what to do! A Pocket Full of Wisdom **2010**

My Destiny arrives on the wings of Triumphant Angels - Just on Time! A Pocket Full of Wisdom **2010**

I am well-poised and divinely inspired. I am creative and Supreme power goes before me and makes my paths straight. A Pocket Full of Wisdom **2010**

I place my requests and petitions before God at the Throne and praise God, my Creator. A Pocket Full of Wisdom **2010**

I make the absolute most and best of opportunities and place my trust in the Supreme to deliver me! A Pocket Full of Wisdom **2010**

Thy kingdom come, Supreme will be done today in all of my ways and dealings!
A Pocket Full of Wisdom **2010**

There is no fear, pain, or anxious thoughts in me. There is only One Infinite Power and there is no Evil. A Pocket Full of Wisdom **2010**

There is no fear, pain, struggle, suffering or anxious thoughts in me; there is only One Infinite Power; God. A Pocket Full of Wisdom **2010**

Evil is nothingness and has no power;
Evil fails to exist! A Pocket Full of
Wisdom **2010**

There is only Good present in my everyday; anything appearing poor is distinguished to absolutely nothing! A Pocket Full of Wisdom **2010**

I'm extremely fortunate and Rich in my private and business dealings and I'm serviced and I'm treated very lavishly, kindly, and respectably. A Pocket Full of Wisdom **2010**

Supreme Power, God's Angels and positive imperceptible forces are ever working for me to increase my love, joy, and prosperity! A Pocket Full of Wisdom **2010**

I treat others very good; likewise, others treat me the best also. A Pocket Full of Wisdom **2010**

My lips are kind, respectful, honorable, loving, and truthful! I am honest, humble, and speak the truth in all necessary situations and circumstances. A Pocket Full of Wisdom **2010**

I aim to see the best in others; likewise others seek to see and perceive the best in me!
A Pocket Full of Wisdom **2010**

I am not wronged and do not wrong others; likewise, I am treated correctly. A Pocket Full of Wisdom **2010**

God sees and knows everything from everlasting to everlasting; I am divinely well mannered and well behaved. A Pocket Full of Wisdom **2010**

Supreme Power moves; but cannot be moved. I move with Supreme grace and any situation or circumstance that is not for me moves away or else I move in Spirit in the correct direction along my way! A Pocket Full of Wisdom **2010**

Supreme Power moves; but cannot be moved! I move amid Supreme grace; any situation or circumstance that is not for me is not present. A Pocket Full of Wisdom **2010**

Supreme Power moves; but cannot be moved! I move amid Spirit in the correct behavior and direction of my destiny! A Pocket Full of Wisdom **2010**

I am not suspicious. Appearances and facades do not concern me; there's no opposition in my game of life. A Pocket Full of Wisdom **2010**

I am not defensive. Appearances are not my concern, so there's no opposition in my game of life. A Pocket Full of Wisdom **2010**

I am a victorious frontrunner, and I move in Powerful Spirit along my way!

A Pocket Full of Wisdom **2010**

I am a favorite choice among men and women to advance their ever-increasing healthy, wealthy, and happy new lives. A Pocket Full of Wisdom **2010**

I am celebrated, inspiring and encouraging in the game of life! A Pocket Full of Wisdom
2010

Love and integrity are key invaluable facets that I bring to every good and worthy situation or circumstance! I possess now the eternal key of True Love and use it wisely as I receive and give Good Godly Love. A Pocket Full of Wisdom **2010**

Well done, good and worthy servant; Infinite Spirit is within me, Thy will be done! A Pocket Full of Wisdom **2010**

God is the Everlasting God of creation and completion; I create and I finish what I am meant to do here on Earth as it is in Heaven. A Pocket Full of Wisdom **2010**

I am victorious! I Celebrate the now and the then! A Pocket Full of Wisdom **2010**

Today is not the "End of Something"; it is the Divine beginning of "Something Better here on Earth as it is in Heaven. *A Pocket Full of Wisdom* **2010**

What is the end, but the beginning of something else? I begin anew, today is a New Beginning... I am Becoming!
A Pocket Full of Wisdom **2010**

Tomorrow is my Dawning; today is my Present! A Pocket Full of Wisdom **2010**

I'm luminous! My Rich Power switch is "On"! A Pocket Full of Wisdom **2010**

I do not labor, whine or complain; Victory is the name of my game! *A Pocket Full of Wisdom* **2010**

I shimmer, illuminate and shine; the infinite victory power is mine! A Pocket Full of Wisdom **2010**

I radiate, sparkle and shimmer; I'm a frontrunner; I am a winner! A Pocket Full of Wisdom **2010**

I establish the Divine Plan upon a rock! No mountain is too hard to climb, no road to narrow or too high, and no slippery slope too steep. I'm grounded and truth is under my feet! A Pocket Full of Wisdom **2010**

Mountains move and tremble at the sound of God's thunder; what God has joined together for me, let no man put asunder! A Pocket Full of Wisdom **2010**

Nothing is subtracted from the vast multiplication of my Riches; increase is added to me. A Pocket Full of Wisdom

2010

God hath coupled together us two and nothing shall be taken away from this joining of two! A Pocket Full of Wisdom **2010**

My love potion number 9 is a 10; I am open and loving and welcome Divine true love in! A Pocket Full of Wisdom **2010**

My Divine Marriage is powerfully and correctly established. I'm grounded, balanced and joined with my correct love! A Pocket Full of Wisdom **2010**

My Divine Rich and pleasurable Business is established. I'm grounded, balanced, happy, healthy, and joined with my correct Business! A Pocket Full of Wisdom **2010**

My Divine Rich and Happy Life is powerfully and correctly established. I'm grounded, balanced and joined with my correct endeavors! A Pocket Full of Wisdom
2010

By the authority vested in me, I now pronounce me, Rich!
Amen.